Acne

How to Cure Acne through Natural Remedies and Simple Habits. Say Goodbye to Pustules, Blackheads and Whiteheads for Good!

Robert S. Lee

Contents

Chapter 1. What Really Causes Your Acne

Acne is a breakout. It's where your skin cells, hair, and even sebum forms a plug in your pore. This plug will then get infected with bacteria, which results in swelling. This forms acne or pimples as the plug starts to break down. Of course, it can be painful, and you need to find a way to get rid of it. Whiteheads are under the skin and are very small, and they're a type of acne, but you also have your blackheads. These are black on the surface of your skin, but they're not caused by dirt. They're clearly visible, though.

Then you have your papules, which are visible on the surface, and they are usually pink and no more than a small bump. You have your pustules, which is clearly visible, and usually they are red with pus at the top. Then your nobules, which are large and solid pimples. They can be painful as they are embedded deep within your skin. You can even form cysts which are a type of acne which usually cause scars. They are usually filled with pus and very painful.

It's Sadly Common:

Acne is sadly very common, and three quarters of people from age eleven to thirteen will get acne at one point. It can affect all people from all walks of life, and it can be difficult, painful, and embarrassing to deal with and get rid of. You don't always need to turn to prescription and over the counter creams and medicine that can be harmful and result in various unpleasant side effects. Instead, it's often best that you use a natural or herbal remedy, which you'll find many in this book.

What Causes It?:

There is no definite answer on what causes acne, but there are many contributing factors, so it is most likely to be a variety of things that have caused your acne overall. For example oily makeup or dirt staying on your face too long can cause acne. Of course, you may also be more prone to acne because of your genetics, but that doesn't mean you can't treat your acne with natural and herbal remedies that help in both the short term and the long term.

You Can Make It Worse:

Remember that squeezing your pimples can actually make acne worse, so popping them isn't usually the best method. Greasy hair can also cause more problems than it's worth. You should also avoid hot and humid climates if you want your acne to start getting better. It'll cause you to sweat more, and sweat can actually make acne worse. This is why you should wash your face more often if you are dealing with acne, but do not leave your skin too dry by over washing or your skin will try to produce more oil to makeup up for it.

You should also try to cut out your anxiety and stress if you're looking to get rid of your acne fast. Anxiety and stress can have a very serious impact on your acne by causing your to secrete more oils, which will clog your pores and cause further breakouts. It can also because you to absent mindedly scratch at your acne, making it worse as well as risking scarring.

Avoid Certain Foods:

Remember that even what you eat can actually cause more acne, so you need to be careful what you're actually eating. There are actually acne trigger foods that should be avoided on top of using natural and herbal remedies. Sadly, on the list is chocolate, as it can be very harmful.

A diet that is high in fat and sugars can cause your body to produce more sebum which promotes inflammation and leads to acne. So you need to cut out the sugary and fatty foods. It's better to eat a diet of fruits and vegetables if you want to have an acne fighting diet, which is also covered in a later chapter. Spicy foods should also be avoided because they can cause sweating and a fluctuation in your hormones, which can lead to acne as well.

Cutting these out of your diet will help you to fight your acne internally. Small changes will add up to help make sure that you're fighting acne internally, and when you use external methods on top of it, you're much more likely to be sure that you're getting rid of your acne for the long term instead of just worrying about the short term.

Chapter 2. Natural Acne Relieving Salves

Salves are a great way to help with acne, and you'll find that it also helps to make sure that you have salves to use in other things as well. Many acne salves will help by doubling as other relief method as well, and they're easy to make so long as you have the right ingredients. Remember that salves often require a larger variety of ingredients, but there are some that are simple. Just find the one that's right for you, and apply it regularly for the best results.

Salve #1 Drawing & Acne Cream

This salve is not just for acne. You can use it for bug bites, and it'll even make more than one batch. It's a black salve, and it can work on boils, splinters, bee stings, infections, and insect bites. Place it on the affected area, and it's usually best to cover it. You'll have a hard time getting it out of clothes, as it does stain.

Ingredients:

1. 9 Teaspoons Olive Oil, Extra Virgin

2. ¼ Cup Plantain Leave

3. ¼ Cup Calendula Flowers

4. ¼ Cup Comfrey Leaves

5. 1 ml Rosemary Extract

6. 1 ml Tea Tree Oil

7. 1 ml Fir Needle Essential Oil

8. 1 ml Lavender Essential Oil

9. 2 ml Vitamin E oil

10. 1 ½ Teaspoon Green Tea Powder

11. 1 ½ Teaspoons Cocoa Butter

12. 1 ½ Teaspoons Extra Virgin Coconut Oil

13. 3 Teaspoons Honey, Raw

14. 3 Teaspoons Beeswax, Raw & Grated

15. 6 Teaspoons Charcoal, Activated

16. 3 Teaspoons Bentonite Clay

Directions:

1. First you're going to want to infuse your oil, and this should be done in advance. Put all of the herbs in a container, and then put the olive oil over it. It will need to sit in a cool, dark location after being sealed for four to six weeks, and you should shake every other day.

2. You can then strain the herbs out of the oil, and you'll have our infused oil. Only use nine teaspoons of it for this recipe, and label the rest and store it in a cool, dark place until you need it again.

3. Take your beeswax and melt it in a double boiler, and then add in your cocoa butter and coconut oil. Stir until melted completely before removing it from heat.

4. Stir your infused oil into the melted mix, adding in the honey.

5. Take your vitamin E oil, rosemary extract, and other essential oils and combine them in a bowl with your green tea powder, activated charcoal and bentonite clay. Make sure it's thoroughly mixed, and then combine it with the

beeswax mix. Make sure it's thoroughly combined all the way through, and then place into glass slave jars for storage.

6. To use put on the area that you're having problems with, and do this at least once daily. Doing it twice daily will result in quicker results.

Salve #2 Thyme Based Acne Cream

Sweet almond is great for dry or irritated skin, but it's also great for acne. It improves your skin health, and it'll help to make sure that you have everything you need to put the thyme essential oil in it. It's a great carrier oil, and thyme essential oil is known to help clear up acne fast. Try to use it at least twice daily.

Ingredients:

1. 2 Teaspoon Baking Soda

2. 1 Teaspoon Sweet Almond Oil

3. 2-4 Drop Thyme Essential Oil

Directions:

1. Mix the essential oil into the sweet almond oil, and then stir it into the baking soda. Make sure to mix completely, and then store it in a label jar.

2. Wash the affected area, and then pat dry before applying the cream. You usually need to add a drop of water, and then let sit for one to three minute. You can then wash anything that hasn't soaked in off.

Salve #3 Rose Soothing Salve

This is more of a gel than a salve, but it's used relatively the same. It's easy to use, and it's even easier to make. You don't have to worry about a complicated ingredient list, and it makes a rather large back that you can store appropriately. Rose even helps to decrease your stress, which may be causing a larger portion of your acne than you're aware of.

Ingredients:

1. 1 Cup Pure Aloe Vera Gel

2. 1 Cup Rose Petals, Fresh & Packed

3. 2-4 Drops Rose Essential Oil

Directions:

1. Just mix everything together, and apply it to the affected area at least once daily.

However, using it two to three times daily will help get rid of your acne faster, and it's even great on sunburns.

Salve #4 Basic Acne Salve

This is an acne salve that uses a basic infused oil, and it only takes a few hours to infuse the oil. The peppermint leave and lavender makes the cream soothing, but the comfrey and plantain leaves are sure to draw out your acne almost immediately. Try to apply twice daily for the best results.

Ingredients:

1. ½ Cup Plantain Leaves

2. ½ Cup Lavender Blossoms, dried

3. ¼ Cup Peppermint Leaves

4. 1 ½ Cups Olive Oil, Extra Virgin

5. 8 Tablespoons Beeswax, Grated

6. ½ Cup Comfrey Leaves

Directions:

1. Infuse the herbs into your oil by cooking the oil over a double boiler for two to three hours. The heat should be on low, and make sure to stir regularly.

2. Strain out the herbs, and then add in a beeswax. It works best if you use it one tablespoon at a time.

3. Place in an airtight container, and store until you need it. Apply gently to the affected area after it's been washed and dried.

Salve #5 Calendula Acne Salve

Calendula is great for acne, and it's a natural herb that's easy to get ahold. Remember to make a large enough batch that you have something to put up, and it'll make making this salve that much easier in the long run. You can use any carrier oil, but sweet almond oil is perfect for glowing healthy skin, which is why it's been added. The lavender is soothing and helps to make sure that your stress is reduced, which is a leading cause of acne. When paired with tea tree oil, your acne will be gone in no time. Like all salves, it works best if you apply twice daily to the affected area after it's been washed in cool water and patted dry.

Ingredients:

1. ¼ Cup Calendula Flowers

2. 1 Cup Sweet Almond Oil

3. 8-10 Drops Lavender Essential Oil

4. 1 Teaspoon Beeswax, Grated

5. 5-6 Drops Tea Tree Oil

6. 2 Tablespoons Coconut Oil

Directions:

1. Start by putting your sweet almond oil and calendula flower in a double boiler,

cooking on low for three hours while stirring. Strain out the herbs, and put in a glass container for storage as an infused calendula oil. Use two tablespoons for this recipe.

2. Melt your beeswax in the double boiler, add in the calendula oil, and your coconut oil. Make sure to stir until completely combined.

3. Add in essential oils, and take off of heat. Place in a glass jar for storage.

Chapter 3. Essential Oils to Help With Bad Acne

Essential oils are also great for acne, but only if you're making sure to use a therapeutic grade essential oil. These are usually a little more expensive, but they're the only ones that will produce results. Remember that you'll need a carrier oil, and coconut oil and sweet almond oil are usually recommended.

Essential Oil #1 Geranium

When you're using a geranium essential oil then acne will be a thing of the past. It can help you to improve your skin, and it even helps with elasticity and to tighten your skin. So it doubles as a way to help make sure that you don't feel the effects of aging. It can heal bruises, cuts, eczema, and other skin conditions. Acne is only one of the issues that geranium oil can help with. Just remember to use it with a carrier oil.

Essential Oil #2 Frankincense

Many people don't think frankincense when they're thinking acne relief, but it's known to help as well. It has anti-inflammatory benefits which are known to help cure up acne quickly. It's usually best when used with a blend, so you'd use only a few drops with another essential oil and a carrier oil together. It can even decrease the appearance of your pores, which will even out skin tone as a natural toner. It can tighten your skin and even reduce the visibility of scars.

Essential Oil #3 Lemon

Lemon essential oil is a little easier and cheaper to get ahold of, which is why it's a common essential oil to use for acne. You don't always have a lot of money to spend, so this is a great essential oil solution. You can always add a few drops to your acne creams, and it's sure to help. It is a natural astringent, and it's even antibacterial. It will help with oily skin, which can often cause acne, and it can reduce the appearance of pores.

Essential Oil #4 Tea Tree

Tea tree essential oil is also something that's easy to get ahold of, and you'll usually find it in your local pharmacy. It can ward of bacteria that usually causes acne, and it can even regulate your oil product. This will decrease your breakouts and the severity of the ones you get. It even has therapeutic qualities, which help you to relieve stress and anxiety, which will also contribute to acne. So say goodbye to acne and to your stress.

Essential Oil #5 Patchouli

If you're dealing with aging and acne, you should make sure that you have patchouli essential oil up your sleeve. It's antibacterial, antifungal and even antiseptic. It will help to make sure your acne, eczema, and wrinkles start to disappear. It'll even help with any fine lines, and psoriasis you may be dealing with. It'll smooth out your face, and it'll help to make sure that everything is right. Of course, it can be used as a main oil in any of your blends.

Essential Oil #6 Oregano

Oregano is a great essential oil, and it's yet another one that isn't that expensive to get and add in to any salve or cream. It's extremely potent and it kills a lot of the bacteria that is response for acne. It can even help your skin to look healthier because it has many vitamin and antioxidants that will help your skin to look younger. You just need two drops of it with ten drops of a carrier oil, and you can apply it topically and directly to the affected area.

Essential Oil #7 Lavender

Lavender is a harder essential oil to get, but it's not too expensive. It's anti-inflammatory and antibacterial, which is great for acne. It can help you to relax, so the stress is gone, and it'll be great at reducing any scars that acne can produce as well. A topical application is all you need, but make sure that you never apply it directly to your skin. Like most essential oils, it can actually harm and irritate your skin if you aren't using a carrier oil. Essential oils are just too strong, especially for sensitive skin.

Essential Oil #8 Bergamot

Bergamot is a great essential oil to use for acne, and it has an extremely pleasant citrus scent as well. It's considered a fragrance that is sure to be revitalizing, and it has antibacterial properties to help to treat any breakout you may be suffering from. It's best in a blend, so don't try to use it on its own if you want the best results. Try to use it with an anti-inflammatory acne treating essential oil, and it'll help to make it a little more powerful. Remember to always use a blend and a carrier oil.

Essential Oil #9 Rosemary

Rosemary isn't that expensive as a therapeutic grade essential oil, and it has a light scent, so it's easy to add in to just about any blend. It revitalizes your skin, and it reduces any excess oil production. It even is anti-inflammatory, and it will help your skin to glow in no time. Add it to any moisturizer or apply it directly to a carrier oil. You can even use it in a blend if you want to. It's a natural astringent, and it'll help to firm and tone your skin as well, making it perfect for anti-aging.

Essential Oil #10 Sandalwood

Sandalwood is a great additive to any acne treatment, and you'll find that it's useful but should never be used as the main essential oil when treating acne. It has some antibacterial and anti-inflammatory effects, but it is not as strong as other essential oils. It adds a great aromatic scent that will help to relax you and relieve stress, so it's great to add, but never as your only oil. It still needs a carrier oil.

Remember:

You shouldn't use essential oils while pregnant unless you have already cleared it with your doctor, and this goes for breast feeding as well. Do not use essential oils on children without permission from your doctor as well, and you need to make sure that all essential oils are blended properly into a carrier oil. Some of the best carrier oils are coconut oil and sweet almond oil. Make sure that you add just a few drops to each teaspoon, and check for skin sensitivity first.

Chapter 4. Remedy Your Problem With the Right Food

Sometimes acne is caused by the food that you're eating, and it can be as simple as making sure that you have the right food. Of course, these dietary changes are often just the start of clearing up your acne. Herbal remedies may still be required, but food can really help by balancing your body. Sometimes acne is because your body is out of balance, as well as stress, and food can help with both of these if you're eating the right things. Remember that sebum production causes your skin to be oily, so it's important that it's regulated and under control if you want your acne to get better in the long term.

Food #1 Blueberries

There's a reason that blueberries are known as a superfood, and you'll find that they can help you with acne as well. Of course, since blueberries are a fruit, most people don't mind adding them into your diet. Fresh is always better, but frozen blueberries will usually do in a pinch. Blueberries are incredibly high in antioxidants, which I going to improve the health of your body overall, but it's also a great way to clear acne flare-ups because it contains pectin, which will clear intestinal toxins. It even has vitamin E which will help to make sure that your skin glows in no time.

Food #2 Carrots

Carrots are great for your eyesight, but they can help you fight acne as well. It's full of beta-carotene, and that converts to vitamin A, which will help with the inflammation that cause acne. It can even regulate your sebum production, which is known to cause problems in your kin a well. You can fight skin and pimples in no time, and it doesn't matter what variety of carrot you use. Just make sure to add it into your diet a little more, but eating them raw always helps a little more.

Food #3 Cilantro

Cilantro is a seasoning, but it's still a great food to help make sure that your acne is well under control. You can easily add this herb into your anti-acne diet, and it is full of vitamin E, which is great for your skin, and it can fight free radicals that will commonly cause damage to your skin, including worsening breakouts. It'll even help because of the beta-carotene that is sure to make sure that you are getting all the anti-inflammatory and anti-microbial properties that cilantro has to offer.

Food #4 Romaine Lettuce

You can add romaine lettuce to your diet to help with any acne flare-ups, and it'll help to stabilize your blood sugar as an added benefit. Vitamin C is great as it helps with the absorption of chromium, which is known to balance out your body as well. You certainly can't reply on it solely to get rid of your acne unless you're eating a salad made of it every day, and even then you may not get enough depending on the severity of your acne breakout, but when you make an acne fighting diet, it's a great addition to add in.

Food #5 Mustard Greens

Mustard greens are also high in beta-carotene, and they'll help to control your sebum production as well to make sure that your skin isn't too oily. It'll also help because of the anti-inflammatory effects, and the vitamin E will have your skin glowing in no time. It has peppery flavor, but it' easy to add in. remember that it'll always work best if you're using it raw, but if you cook it it'll still help as well.

Food #6 Barley

Barley is a little easier to add into your diet than mustard greens for most people, and it won't affect your blood sugar levels that badly. If you have excess insulin in your blood stream, then you'll find that it can increase your androgen circulation sharply, which is associated with acne breakouts. You can't use it if you're allergic to gluten or at least sensitive to them, so make sure that you add barley into your next soup to get some acne fighting benefits. It's even a cheap ingredient.

Food #7 Almonds

Almonds are a great snack, and they can help you maintain a healthy weight, lose weight, and even help with your acne breakouts. It's because they're high in selenium, and it's a powerful antioxidants that will reduce inflammation as well as help with skin elasticity. This will help to make sure that you get clearer skin quickly, and you can either cook with them or just eat a handful a day for a snack. You can even put them in your lunch or breakfast. They're easy to pack, and they give you the selenium intake you need.

Food #8 Oranges

Fruit is always easy to add into your diet, and you'll find the reason that oranges should be added into your acne fighting diet is because of its high vitamin C content. For this reason spinach, tomatoes, or even melons will usually work as well. When you strengthen the walls of your cells and your immune system with vitamin C, you're going to help your body repair damaged and irritated skin. This helps you to get rid of your acne breakout that much faster.

Food #9 Green Tea

Green tea is more of a drink than a food, but it's a drink that is easy to add into any acne fighting diet. Of course, you'll find that you can sweeten it with honey if you want added results because honey and green tea both have a large amount of antioxidants. It will help to protect your skin from damage and breakouts, and it'll help to add it to your daily routine. It can even help to make sure that that you relax during the day, as green tea can help with stress, and honey has been known to be helpful as well.

Food #10 Brown Rice

Brown rice is actually extremely helpful in acne fighting as well, and that's because it is high in magnesium. Magnesium will balance hormones that are acne-inducing, and many people have a magnesium deficiency. Even if you don't, it won't hurt to give yourself a magnesium boost, and you can even use artichoke, oatmeal and figs to help make sure that you're getting the magnesium you need.

Chapter 5. Natural Supplements to Help with Acne

There are many supplements that you can take for acne as well, and supplements are the way to go for natural acne relief for many people. Remember that a supplement won't work miracles, but it will help to make sure that you're getting your body back into balance, which will help to make sure that you lessen your chances of a breakout. Of course, if you're already in the middle of one, you won't just be able to get rid of it quickly with supplements. Supplements are much more of a long term solution, but they don't provide immediate results.

Supplement #1 Vitamin A

Vitamin A is a great supplement to take if you're looking to help with acne. Vitamin A is antioxidant rich, and contains retinol, which is known to help with acne. You can take it orally as a supplement, and it'll help with inflammation which often causes acne, and it can clear up your skin, and it has the added benefit of boosting your immune system and helping to improve your vision or keeping it at a normal level. With vitamin A you won't have to worry so much about shedding the dead skin cells that will block your pores and cause acne. It'll keep your pores from clogging, and it'll calm any breakout.

Supplement #2 Zinc

Zinc is also great at fighting acne and that's because it assists with the metabolism of omega-3 fatty acids. It helps your body to absorb them, and this supplements helps by giving you the antioxidants your skin needs to fight off breakouts, as well as having anti-inflammatory properties which is known to help as well. It even transports vitamin A, helping the vitamin A you're taking to work. Zinc is a great supplement if you're already on an acne fighting diet because it'll help other vitamins to get into your body and help fight acne as well.

Supplement #3 Omega-3 Fatty Acids

Omega-3 fatty acids are also great at fighting acne, and you may not be getting enough from your regular diet. Adding it in as a supplement is a great way to help. It inhibits two chemicals that cause inflammation, which can cause your acne as well. You'll find that inflammation is one of the main reasons for acne, and that' because it clogs your pores. You'll find that if you're consuming enough omega-3 you will have a lesser chance of developing acne.

Supplement #4 Selenium

Selenium is great for an acne fighting diet, and it's great as a supplement if you think you're not getting enough as well. It helps to preserve levels of zinc an antioxidants, and it can prevent inflammation, which helps as well. It works great with vitamin E, and if you're deficient in selenium, then you're much more likely to have psoriasis, acne breakouts, and eczema. It should be taken along with antioxidants in your diet for the bet results.

Supplement #5 Turmeric

Turmeric is a common spice, and it's used in Indian cuisine. You may actually find it's already in your spice cabinet, but it should also be in your supplements. Turmeric is anti-inflammatory, and it's known to work wonders. It helps to treat acne because of the high amount of anti-inflammatory properties. It's easy to get, and you can get Turmeric or curcumin, which will both help. Many supplements actually mix the two, and it'll help to provide long term relief from acne breakouts.

Supplement #6 Green Tea Extract

Acne is commonly caused by inflammation and hormonal imbalances, which the antioxidants offered in green tea extract can help with. Green tea is a supplement that has an incredibly high amount of green antioxidants. You can of course use green tea in your anti-acne diet, but if you don't like the taste, then the green tea extract is considered to be a great addition to any supplements you may be taking.

Supplement #7 Vitamin B5

This is a vitamin that some people say will work and many others say won't. However, for some people it really does. Of course, many people have to take the highest dose per day that their doctor allows to get rid of it quickly. Otherwise, it' just going to work in the long run. It's something you should always ask your doctor about before taking due to the high amount of vitamin B5 that is necessary to help clear up your acne. It's best to add with antioxidants for the best result. You may have a vitamin B5 deficiency, which commonly will contribute to acne breakouts.

Supplement #8 Milk Thistle

Your liver is extremely important, and if you're suffering from acne you may have a sluggish liver that needs a boost. Without your liver working at top speed, there will be many toxins in your body and you won't be regulating your hormones like you should, which can cause acne. With your hormones regulated and toxins being pumped out of your system instead of staying around, you're much less likely to suffer from bad acne breakouts.

Supplement #9 Fermented Cod Liver Oil

There are many nutrients in fermented cod liver oil, and it can contribute easily to your overall skin and health. It will help you absorb Omega-3 fatty acids, K2, vitamin D, and even vitamin A. it can even help your brain and immune system. Of course, it's great for hormonal imbalances, which will commonly cause your breakout. It is great for your skin.

Remember:

You shouldn't take any supplements without talking to your doctor first, and list any over the counter medication you may be taking as well.

Supplements can interact with prescription medication, herbal remedies, and over the counter medication like any other medications. You should never take any supplement while pregnant or breastfeeding unless you've cleared it with your doctor. Always make sure that you are using supplements with an acne fighting diet and creams for the best results. You can have allergic reactions to supplements like any other medication, and you should look out for any signs of an allergic reaction or side effects.

Chapter 6. Herbal Facemasks to Help

Herbal facemasks and scrubs are great at helping to make sure that you get results quickly. Relief from acne is important to your self-esteem and confidence, and getting rid of it is important if you want to feel more confident about yourself. With the right herbal facemasks or scrub, then you'll find that your acne can clear up within a matter of days.

Facemask #1 Simple 2 Ingredient Facemask

Sometimes you don't want to have to buy too many ingredients and this facemask is great for that. You'll need to order your bentonite clay, but other than that apple cider vinegar is easy to get ahold of. Bentonite clay is great at making sure that your face clears up, and apple cider vinegar will help to clean out your pores, and it's antibacterial.

Ingredients:

1. ½ Cup Bentonite Clay

2. ½ Cup Apple Cider Vinegar

Directions:

1. Mix together, and store in a glass container.

2. When using, make sure that the area is clean and patted dry. Then apply the facemask, allowing it to sit for fifteen to twenty minutes before washing off with cool water.

Facemask #2 Honey & Lemon Mask

Honey is great for moisturizing skin, and it makes your skin look younger almost immediately. Of course, lemon is antibacterial, and it'll help to make sure that any bacteria that might be causing your acne to flare up.

Ingredients:

1. 1 Teaspoon Lemon Juice, Fresh

2. 2-3 Drops Frankincense Essential Oil

3. 1 Teaspoon Honey, Raw

Directions:

1. Mix everything together, and apply it to the area. Make sure to let it dry on for ten to fifteen minutes.

2. Wash clean with cool water, and pat dry.

Facemask #3 Turmeric Mask

Turmeric is great for your skin, and you'll find that it'll help when applied topically as well. It helps with dry skin, withered skin, and it helps with moisturizing and slowing down aging. It can even make your skin a little more firm, and the honey and milk is a great moisturizer to help your skin glow as it's cleared from its acne breakout quickly and effectively.

Ingredients:

1. ¼ Teaspoon Turmeric Powder

2. 1 ½ Teaspoons Honey, Raw

3. 1 Teaspoon Milk, Whole & Chilled

Directions:

1. Make sure to remove any makeup first, and gently wash your face. This will help to open up your pores. Once your face is dry, mix all the ingredients together in a bowl.

2. Apply to the affected area, and let it sit for eight to twelve minutes. It should dry completely, and then you can rinse off with cool water.

Facemask #4 Honey & Spice Mask

If you're looking for a facemask that also smells great, then you've found it. It's made with cinnamon and nutmeg, which is great at detoxing your skin and helping to make sure that it repairs itself from any breakout. It's even anti-inflammatory and antibacterial, helping to get rid of your breakout quickly. It even has antioxidants thanks to the raw honey used in this facemask recipe.

Ingredients:

1. 3 Tablespoons Honey, Raw

2. ½ Teaspoon Cinnamon, Ground

3. ¼ Teaspoon Nutmeg, Ground

Directions:

1. Mix everything together, and after washing and drying your face you'll want to apply it to the affected area.

2. Wait ten to fifteen minutes before you rinse off with cool water.

Facemask #5 Green Tea Facemask Blend

Green tea is great for your skin due to the antioxidants, and you'll find that when it's applied to your face it can work just as well if not better than if you're taking it internally. Lemon juice is also great at fighting acne because it is antibacterial, helping to reduce any bacteria that is worsening your breakout.

Ingredients:

1. 1 ½ Teaspoon Matcha Powder

2. 1 ½ Tablespoon Lemon Juice, Fresh

Directions:

1. Mix together and apply to the area. Let it sit for ten to fifteen minutes before rinsing off with cool water.

Facemask #6 Strawberry Mask

Many people love the scent of strawberries, and they can be applied topically to your face to help with acne as well. They have alicylic acid, and this is used in a variety of acne products. It can address the bacteria that is causing your acne, and the Greek yogurt helps to sooth and moisturize your skin.

Ingredients:

1. 2 Tablespoons Greek Yogurt, Original

2. ¼ Cup Strawberries, Fresh

Directions:

1. Blend your strawberries into a puree, and then add your Greek yogurt in. make sure it's mixed well.

2. Apply to the affected area, and then let it sit for fifteen to twenty minutes before washing clean.

Facemask #7 Avocado & Honey Mask

Avocado is great to purify your pores, and it can cleanse your face, helping to clean your pores out and make your acne disappear. Of course, you need honey to help with hydration, and it'll help due to its antioxidants as well.

Ingredients:

1. ½ Avocado, Peeled & Cubed

2. 2 Tablespoons Honey, Raw

Directions:

1. Place your avocado cubes in a blender, and blend with honey.

2. Wash the affected area, and apply. Let it sit for fifteen to twenty minutes, and then wash clean with cool water.

Facemask #8 Tomatoes & Greek Yogurt Mask

Tomatoes are rich in vitamin A, and it's going to help with your skin health. It can help with acne as well as acne cars, and it'll reduce the appearance of scars after only a few applications. Greek yogurt will help to make sure your pores are clear, moisturized and glowing. You can use this facemask no matter the severity of your breakout, and it's easy to make.

Ingredients:

1. 1 Tomato, Medium

2. 2 Tablespoons Greek Yogurt

Directions:

1. Cut your tomato into chunk, and then you can put it in a blender, blending with the Greek yogurt.

2. After cleaning your face, apply and let it sit for ten to fifteen minutes. Then you can wash off with cool water.

Chapter 7. Herbal Body Scrubs that Work

Sometimes you need to use something to get rid of acne on your entire body, and it's much easier to use a premade scrub. It even makes a great gift, and when done right they smell amazing. Acne scrubs are easy to make, and the difficulty depends on the scrub you use. Just make them in advance and store them. Just scrub your skin down with it, and then wash away. Use it whenever you're in the shower.

Body Scrub #1 Cinnamon & Vanilla

Cinnamon is antibacterial, and you'll find that vanilla is soothing and reduces stress. It's also anti-inflammatory, which is especially effective when you're using the essential oil. If you don't have cinnamon essential oil add another half teaspoon of cinnamon powder, and if you don't have vanilla essential oil, then add a teaspoon of vanilla extract. However, these substitutes won't be as helpful as the essential oils in treating your acne, but they'll still help.

Ingredients:

1. 1 Tablespoon Cinnamon Powder

2. 2-3 Drops Cinnamon Essential Oil

3. 5-8 Drops Vanilla Essential Oil

4. ½ Cup Coconut Oil

5. 1 Cup White Sugar

Directions:

1. Mix together, and then put in an airtight glass container, and store until you want to use it.

Body Scrub #2 Oatmeal Scrub

You can make your oatmeal scrub in advance or you can put enough of it up to use long term. Of course, make sure that you replace it every two to three weeks, and keep in a cool dark place. Many people will keep it in the fridge, and it helps to make it last. Oatmeal is great at brightening your skin, and honey is antibacterial and has a lot of antioxidants that are sure to help. The olive oil will also help with your skin.

Ingredients:

1. 1 Cup Oatmeal

2. 6 Tablespoons Honey, Raw

3. 3 Tablespoons Olive Oil

Directions:

1. Mix together and put it up until you're ready to use it.

Body Scrub #3Sweet Lemon

Lemon is antibacterial and it's great at treating acne. Add a little vanilla and just a few drops of cinnamon essential oil, and you'll have a fragrant blend that's sure to treat the inflammation, bacteria, and help with stress that can cause acne. It's even known to brighten your mood.

Ingredients:

1. ¾ Cup White Sugar

2. ¼ Cup Sea Salt, Fine

3. 1 Small Lemon, Squeezed

4. ½ Cup Coconut Oil

5. 4-5 Drops Cinnamon Essential Oil

6. 5-8 Drops Vanilla Essential Oil

Directions:

1. Mix all ingredients together, and store appropriately.

Body Scrub #4 Lavender Body Scrub

Lavender essential oil is great for acne, and it can even help with any stress that you may be experiencing. Your acne and stress can be a thing of the past in no time, and it can help with sun spots, acne, cell regeneration, and carrot seed oil is also great for cell regeneration. It'll even help with keeping your skin tone.

Ingredients:

1. ½ Cup Almond Oil

2. 10-15 Drops Lavender Essential Oil

3. 4-5 Drops Carrot Seed Essential Oil

4. 1 Cup Sea Salt, Medium Fine

Directions:

1. Mix all ingredients together, and then use when desired.

Body Scrub #5 Coconut Oil & Turmeric

Coconut oil is great for skin, and it'll help you get glowing skin that's moisturized. With honey you have wonderful antioxidants, and the turmeric and cinnamon powder will help with bacteria and inflammation that may be causing your acne.

Ingredients:

1. 1 Cup Sea Salt, Coarse

2. ½ Cup Coconut Oil

3. 4 Tablespoons Turmeric

4. 5-6 Drops Cinnamon Essential Oil

Directions:

1. Mix together and apply as necessary.

Body Scrub #6 Super Scrub Blend

From the lavender essential oil which helps to clear up your skin and tone it, to the frankincense essential oil that helps with bacteria and inflammation, your acne will be a thing of the past. Add in honey and lemon juice, and you have a wonderful sugar scrub that should help anywhere on your body, and the almond oil is perfect for making your skin glow.

Ingredients:

1. 1 Cup White Sugar

2. 5-8 Drops Lavender Essential Oil

3. 2 Tablespoons Lemon Juice, Fresh

4. 3 Tablespoons Honey, Raw

5. 10-12 Drops Frankincense Essential Oil

Directions:

1. Mix everything together, and use as necessary. Place in a cool, dark place for storage.

Body Scrub #7 Green Tea & Vanilla

Green tea is full of antioxidants, and the vanilla is great for uplifting your mood. Many people underestimate how much stress cause acne, and you can get your mood balanced out. The antioxidants are sure to help, and it can help with the effects of aging as well.

Ingredients:

1. 1 Cup White Sugar

2. 6 Tablespoons Green Tea Powder

3. 8-10 Drops Vanilla Essential Oil

4. 2-4 Drops Peppermint Essential Oil

5. ½ Cup Sweet Almond Oil

Directions:

1. Make sure to mix everything together, and store in an airtight glass jar in a cool, dark place.

Chapter 8. Acne Bonus Tips to Help

There are still many tips that you can enjoy to help you get rid of your acne, and you don't have to rely just on a simple scrub to do it. A lot of your lifestyle can be contributing to your acne, so it's important to be careful what you're doing and putting into your body if you want your acne to go away in the long term.

Tip #1 Sunscreen is Important

Sunscreen really helps you look younger, and it'll help you to keep wrinkles away. It'll also keep your skin from getting damaged, which will actually promote a breakout. If it helps with premature aging, then it's a sunscreen that is going to help make sure that you aren't making your breakouts worse or getting a breakout at all.

Tip #2 Clean All Makeup Brushes

If you are one of those women who rarely or never washes their sponges and brushes, then bacteria is breeding there. It can actually cause a breakout, and it's important that you wash your makeup brushes and sponges every other week. If you're using it for foundation, make sure to wash it at least once a week. If you aren't using foundation, then your brushes will actually need to be washed out once a week or more. You can use a shampoo in a cup of water. Just a few drop will do it. Then use it to clean, rinse, and then pat dry. Make sure to let them air dry the rest of the way before using them again.

Tip #3 Get Enough Sleep

Getting enough sleep is also important for controlling your acne breakouts. Your body can't renew its cells if you aren't sleeping right because most of the renewal happens while you're asleep. Sleep deprivation can cause you to have outbreaks, wrinkles and a pale and washed out appearance. So make sure that you're going to bed at a timely manner and waking up feeling refreshed and well rested.

Tip #4 Clean Your Makeup Off Before You Sleep

You need to clean all of your makeup off before you go to sleep if you want to avoid acne breakouts. If you don't, then you're going to clog your pores. It can even cause dryness that is damaging to your skin. It's important to remove your makeup thoroughly, including your eye makeup. You don't want any bumpy rashes or acne coming up. An oil-free cleanser is usually best, especially if you're using waterproof makeup.

Tip #5 Stay Hydrated No Matter What

Hydration matters, especially when it comes to your skin, so make sure that you're drinking the water you need. If you're dehydrated it can actually cause acne breakouts. This is because your skin is going to try to produce more oil because it's dry. This can turn into a breakout, but drinking water is really an easy solution.

Tip #6 Wash Before & After Workouts

It's important to wash your face before and after workouts. You don't want makeup while you're working out because it'll mix with the sweat, which will result in clogging your pores. You'll also want to get the sweat off your face and hydrate it after workout if you want to avoid an acne breakout later on.

Tip #7 Change Your Pillowcases Regularly

Many people don't think about trying to change their pillowcases more often, but it's important if you're suffering from acne. Your hair often clings onto oil, and you'll find that if you aren't changing your pillowcases then you're sleeping on oil all night long. It can be avoided by making sure that your pillowcases are clean so the oil isn't there and just accumulating.

Tip #8 Workout More Often

You'll find that working out can actually help to decrease acne. It's because stress can cause a lot of flare ups, but it's reduced when you're working out. It's important to work out daily if you want it to help you with general acne breakouts, and it's easy to do. Just try to work out for thirty minutes every day, and your acne should improve.

Tip #9 Stop Touching Your Face

If you are having issues with breakouts on your face, then you really need to stop touching your face for the best result, especially if you're using natural creams and scrubs. Your fingers are oily, and they have dirt you aren't seeing. This is getting on your skin and clogging your pores. You don't need to add that to your acne prone skin, so keep your hands off your face if you want to reduce the amount of breakouts that you usually get.

Tip #10 Avoid Oil Based Makeup

Oil based makeup is probably the worst makeup you can buy for yourself, especially if you're struggling with acne. It'll clog your pores, and that's sure to actually harm your pores and cause inflammation. Just skip the oil based products and go for something a little lighter. It'll make a large difference.

Remember:

You need to be patient with any product that you're using. You won't clear up your acne overnight, so you need to make sure that you're giving yourself the time to clear your acne. Combining scrubs, herbal supplements, and facemasks is really going to help with your acne, especially if you're using an acne fighting diet as well. Give it time, and you're sure to find a natural acne remedy that is sure to work for you.